TABLE OF CONTENTS

I0421056

INTRODUCTION

While men and women have many of the same health problems, they can affect women differently. For example, women are more likely to die after a heart attack than men are. Women suffer greater rates of depression and osteoarthritis affects more women than men.

A woman's body is different than a man's in more ways than the obvious and so they have special needs that drive reasons to gain awareness, and take action in prevention in the hope of reducing risk factors for various conditions.

Too often in this ultra hectic modern world, women tend to neglect self-care until it's too late. Today, women work, and take care of a household and children, which often leaves little time for them.

Taking the time to become aware of common health threats, and lifestyle choices that can improve health and wellbeing is not only recommended, it is necessary to ensure good health even into old age.

Welcome To Your Health!

*"If you think taking care of yourself is selfish, change your mind.
If you don't, you're simply ducking your responsibilities."*
~ Ann Richards

Surprisingly, men and women have the same hormones inside their bodies—just in different amounts. While the hormonal milieu of men stays about the same over time, women have wide fluctuations in their reproductive hormones according to their menstrual cycle. Postmenopausal women return to a state where the hormones fluctuate little, if at all.

As children, women have ovaries that are relatively nonfunctional. They make very little estrogen and progesterone and almost no testosterone. When puberty happens, the cycle of female hormones begins and the levels of estrogen, progesterone, follicle stimulating hormone, and luteinizing hormone fluctuate with the menstrual cycle.

The Cycle

1. The pituitary gland secretes FSH (follicle stimulating hormone) and LH (luteinizing hormone) in response to signaling from the hypothalamus in the brain.

2. The LH and FSH levels peak at ovulation, causing an egg to be released from among several partially developing eggs in the ovaries. This LH peak is what is measured on home ovulation test strips.

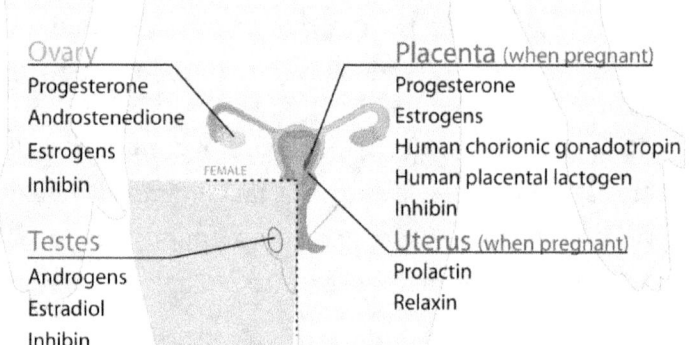

Ovary
Progesterone
Androstenedione
Estrogens
Inhibin

FEMALE

Testes
Androgens
Estradiol
Inhibin

Placenta (when pregnant)
Progesterone
Estrogens
Human chorionic gonadotropin
Human placental lactogen
Inhibin

Uterus (when pregnant)
Prolactin
Relaxin

3. When the ovary releases an egg, the cyst in which the egg was created begins to make progesterone and this level is elevated for about two weeks.

4. If the egg isn't fertilized, the estrogen and progesterone level falls off and the progesterone level remains low until the next ovulation has occurred. Estrogen fluctuates less but is also made in the ovaries and helps to develop the growing egg.

Three Kinds of Estrogen

Three kinds of estrogen are produced in the female body:

- **Estradiol** - main estrogen produced by menstruating women
- **Estriol** - type of estrogen commonly seen in pregnancy although it is made in small amounts at other times
- **Estrone** - type of estrogen produced by postmenopausal women

Women's ovaries (and adrenal glands) make testosterone, too, but in lesser amounts than is seen in males. It is the testosterone in the female system that is responsible for the female sex drive and is why the female sex drive isn't as strong as it is in men.

THE FEEDBACK LOOP

The hormones of the female body are involved in a careful feedback loop that relies on the functioning of the ovaries, the hypothalamus, and the pituitary gland. If any of these are off, the cycle gets out of control and the normal pattern of ovulation does not occur.

During the first half of the menstrual cycle, the estradiol in a woman's system causes the eggs to mature and is why the uterine lining thickens during that time. It is all in preparation for the possibility of a fertilized egg to have a place to rest after ovulation. Because the estrogen level is up, a feedback loop keeps the LH and FSH low.

At the time of ovulation, the pituitary gland releases a burst of LH and FSH in order to allow the release of the egg. Progesterone levels keep the egg supported until it can be fertilized and begins to make its own progesterone. The window of opportunity for fertilization is actually fairly narrow, just a couple of days. The progesterone blocks the LH, which goes back down and the progesterone begins to change the uterine lining in further preparation for the possibility of a fertilized egg implanting in the uterus.

If the egg is fertilized, the levels of progesterone and estrogen remain high to support the uterine lining and the zygote (tiny embryo) to implant in the uterine lining. The implanted zygote makes HCG, which supports the entire system throughout the pregnancy. HCG (human chorionic gonadotropin) is the "pregnancy hormone" that is detected in home pregnancy tests.

If the egg is not fertilized, the progesterone and estrogen levels plummet, causing the uterine lining to escape the body during the menstrual period.

It is all a very complex system that must rely on activity of several endocrine glands in order to work properly. A woman has only so many eggs in her lifetime, and when they "run out," a woman goes through menopause and the ovary puts out much less estrogen, progesterone and testosterone, so that the postmenopausal woman's sex drive diminishes and she no longer has stimulation of the uterine lining. This is when periods stop.

After menopause, the hormone levels do not fluctuate and the FSH levels and LH levels from the pituitary gland are not released in a cyclical fashion any more.

HOW HORMONES INTERACT

Many women wonder why, when one thing goes wrong, such as when they have a low thyroid condition, it affects things like the reproductive system, weight, and energy levels - all at the same time. This is because our endocrine system is tightly interconnected, with feedback loops and multiple uses for some hormones so that it takes the entire functioning system to feel better.

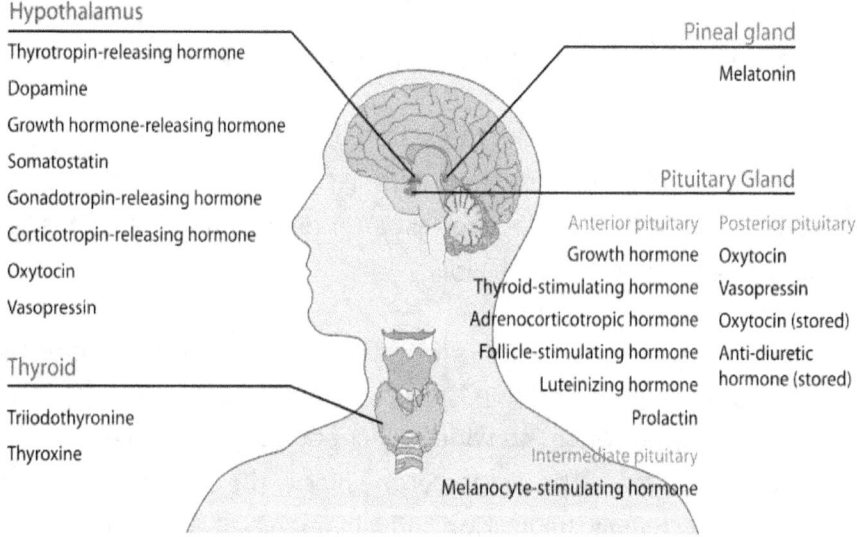

The Pituitary Gland: The Master Gland

The pituitary gland is a tiny gland about the size of a small marble, located at the bottom of the hypothalamus in the brain. The hypothalamus strongly affects the pituitary gland, making a direct connection with hormones that cause the pituitary gland to function. Without the pituitary gland, attached to the hypothalamus by a slender stalk, many endocrine functions do not work. You'll see in a minute why this is the case.

The hypothalamus is located just above the brain stem. It takes in stimuli from the entire peripheral nervous system and helps regulate our blood pressure, temperature, hormone, water, and nutrient concentration. Sometimes the hypothalamus acts on its own but it's most important function in the endocrine system is to make and release hormones that act directly on the pituitary gland, which is called the "Master Gland" because of all of the functions it does.

The pituitary gland is made of two lobes: the anterior lobe and the posterior lobe. The anterior pituitary gland makes the bulk of the hormones, which in turn causes peripheral glands of the body to release or hold back on the making of still other hormones.

The hypothalamus and pituitary gland, along with the peripheral glands of the body, act inside a feedback loop so that when enough hormones are in the body, the pituitary gland shuts down so as not to stimulate the peripheral glands until hormone levels drop again.

This is all tightly regulated so you need every gland to work properly for the feedback loops to work.

The hypothalamus secretes both inhibiting hormones and releasing hormones, which are delivered to the pituitary gland through tiny blood vessels located along the stalk that connects the two structures. The pituitary gland then releases various tropic hormones that cause peripheral glands to take action.

The two hormones released by the pituitary gland are antidiuretic hormone (ADH) and oxytocin.

- Antidiuretic hormone is the hormone that regulates fluid and electrolyte balance in the body.
- Oxytocin is the hormone that causes uterine contractions during labor. It also helps with milk secretion during lactation.

Hormones Released By The Hypothalamus

The hormones released by the hypothalamus help the pituitary gland function. Abnormalities of the hypothalamus can severely affect the function of all glands of the body:

- Growth hormone releasing hormone causes the release of growth hormone from the anterior pituitary gland.
- Somatostatin causes the inhibition of growth hormone release from the anterior pituitary gland.
- Thyrotropin releasing hormone stimulates the release of TSH from the anterior pituitary gland, which in turn causes the thyroid gland to release its own hormones, T3 and T4.
- Gonadotropin releasing hormone causes the anterior pituitary gland to release LH and FSH, which are reproductive hormones acting on both the male and female gonads.

- Prolactin releasing hormone causes the anterior pituitary gland to release prolactin during lactation.
- Dopamine inhibits the release of prolactin by the pituitary gland.
- Corticotropin releasing hormone causes the anterior pituitary gland to release ACTH, which then causes the adrenal gland to release cortisol.

In the anterior pituitary gland, there is the release of thyroid stimulating hormone commonly referred to as TSH, which stimulates the thyroid gland, ACTH, which stimulates cortisol release from the adrenal gland, luteinizing hormone or LH, which causes ovulation and increases testosterone levels, and follicle stimulating hormone or FSH that induces the production of eggs and sperm, depending on whether you are female or male.

As mentioned, the anterior pituitary gland also secretes prolactin and growth hormone, which stimulate milk production and growth, respectively.

The Peripheral Glands

The peripheral glands are where all the action is. This is where the hormones are released that act directly on the cells of the body. For example, when the TSH in the pituitary gland is released, it triggers the release of thyroxine (T4) and triiodothyronine (T3) from the thyroid gland, which regulate the metabolism of all the cells of the body.

The thyroid gland also releases calcitonin, which regulates the amount of calcium and phosphorus in the body. If the T4 and T3 are too low, it sends a feedback signal to release more TSH from the pituitary gland to try and further stimulate the thyroid gland.

The parathyroid glands, located deep within the thyroid gland, causes the release of parathyroid hormone (PTH), which increases the calcium content in the body.

Stress Hormones

The adrenal glands are also very important. They are located on top of each kidney and release cortisol (stress hormone), which increase glucose levels and cause changes in the body related to stress.

They also release aldosterone, which regulate sodium and fluid balance in the kidneys. Deep within the adrenal glands, the adrenal medulla secretes epinephrine and norepinephrine, which are important hormones in the body's "fight or flight" response, occurring under stress.

They increase heart rate, blood pressure, and respiratory rate, shunting blood from the core of the body to peripheral muscles where they can better "fight" or "flee" from perceived danger.

Other Hormones

The male and female gonads produce the hormones that make us have male and female characteristics. For example, the ovaries release estrogen and progesterone, which prepares the birth canal during childbirth.

The ovaries also release inhibin, which turns off the FSH production in the pituitary gland. Estrogen and progesterone act on the uterine wall to stimulate and mature the uterine lining. In males, the testicles produce testosterone, which increases libido, aids in sperm production, and give men the traditional male characteristics. The testes also release inhibin, which turns off FSH production in males.

The pancreas is also partly an endocrine gland, releasing glucagon to raise blood sugar and insulin to lower blood sugar. It also releases somatostatin and pancreatic polypeptide, which act on growth hormone and regulate the release of insulin and glucagon.

The pineal gland is located within the skull. It releases melatonin in response to the absence or presence of light and helps us feel sleepy when it gets dark out and is time to go to bed.

The kidneys also release hormones. For example, erythropoietin stimulates the formation of more red blood cells from the bone marrow. It also releases calcitriol, which acts on the small intestines to increase the serum calcium absorption.

How It All Fits Together

The various glands and hormones are all interconnected. If, for example, the ovaries don't work, it triggers FSH and LH from the pituitary gland, which tries to further stimulate ovarian production of hormones.

- In women, the levels of all the reproductive hormones and reproductive-related pituitary hormones fluctuate with the menstrual cycle and are responsible for the maturation of the uterine lining, the egg, and for the presence of the menstrual period if an egg is not fertilized.
- During menopause, the ovaries cease production of estrogen, progesterone, and testosterone (the actual amounts are not zero but are very low when compared to the childbearing years) and there is no cyclical variation in the levels of the various hormones.

Many of the hormones have feedback loops to make sure that the hormone levels stay at the right levels. If the pituitary gland fails, many other bodily functions fail as well.

On the other hand, if one of the peripheral glands fails, only those functions of the gland are inhibited.

Overactive peripheral glands or an overactive pituitary gland can create a host of symptoms, depending on which glands and hormone levels are affected.

PMS AND PMDD

The LH hormone surge occurs during ovulation as the egg is released and the ovary creates a large amount of estrogen and progesterone in the last half of the menstrual cycle is when many women experience hormonal changes consistent with premenstrual syndrome.

It is possible for any woman to develop mood changes during the last half of the cycle but some experience mood changes so significant that it interferes with daily life, and this may mean a condition known as Premenstrual Dysphoric Disorder or PMDD.

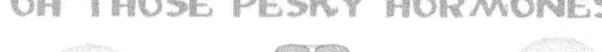

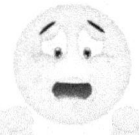
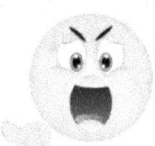
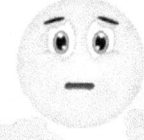
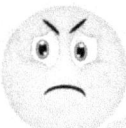

PMDD Symptoms:

- Severe mood swings that can change by the day or hour
- Sadness, loneliness, and hopelessness
- Increased anger
- Anxiety
- Loss of interest in hobbies and regular activities
- Irritability
- Problems with concentration
- Sleepiness or fatigue during the day
- An increase or decrease in appetite
- Insomnia
- Feeling out of control or overwhelmed by life's challenges
- Breast tenderness, bloating, headaches, joint pain, and muscle pain

These symptoms can interfere with daily functioning and affect a woman's relationships both at work and at home.

Vitamins, a healthy diet, and regular exercise can help. If the symptoms are severe, a doctor may suggest other effective treatments that can include oral contraceptives or even prescription medication.

THYROID HEALTH

Women have a greater risk for low thyroid conditions when compared to men. This is partly because they have a higher incidence of autoimmune diseases such as Hashimoto thyroiditis and a higher incidence of Grave's disease.

Women who have low thyroid conditions, also called hypothyroidism, often suffer from obesity, constipation, fatigue, dry skin and a low metabolism. This is because we need the hormones (thyroxine and triiodothyronine) made by the thyroid gland in order to boost cellular metabolism in all cells of the body.

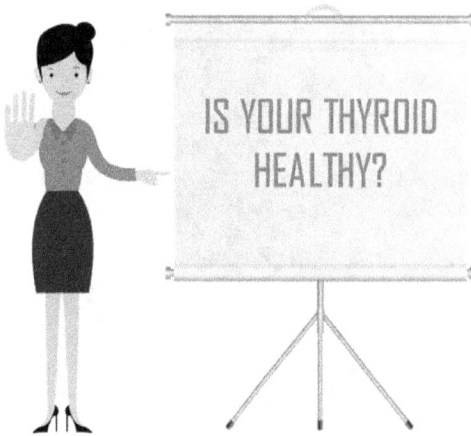

Women especially should see their doctor and have their thyroid hormones checked periodically, including the level of thyroid stimulating hormone or TSH, which is the hormone produced by the pituitary gland whenever the levels of thyroid hormone are too low. A high level of TSH is actually a better measurement of a low thyroid condition than are the measurements of thyroid hormones, T3 and T4.

DIET FOR THYROID HEALTH

Women need a healthy thyroid gland to maintain an elevated metabolism and to keep the weight down. Foods, which help keep the thyroid healthy, include the following:

- **Fish:** Fish are high in omega 3 fatty acids, particularly fatty fish like trout, wild salmon, sardines, and tuna. Omega 3 fatty acids decrease levels of inflammation, improve the immunity, and help increase the levels of selenium, important for thyroid function.
- **Whole grains:** Whole grains help reduce the symptoms of constipation in women who have hypothyroidism. Unfortunately, it binds to exogenous sources of thyroid hormone (thyroid supplements) and can lessen their effectiveness. Take your thyroid supplements on an empty stomach or whenever you are not eating whole grains.
- **Nuts:** Nuts contain a great deal of selenium, which help the thyroid gland work better. Because nuts are high in fat and calories, they should be eaten in moderation.
- **Fresh vegetables and fruits:** These great low calorie foods keep you from gaining weight if your thyroid function is lower than normal. Eat those fruits and vegetables highest in iodine. A diet low in iodine can contribute to goiter and low thyroid function.
- **Seaweed:** Seaweed contains a lot of iodine, a necessary part of thyroid function. Iodine is essential for the making of T4 and T3 in the thyroid gland. If you don't have access to seaweed or don't like it, get your iodine through the taking of iodized salt. Iodized salt has decreased the incidence of iodine-related goiter since it was introduced to the public. Too much iodine, however, can make thyroid disease worse.
- **Dairy products:** Dairy products are high in vitamin D. Low levels of vitamin D appear to increase the risk of Hashimoto's thyroiditis, which is the most common type of hypothyroidism.
- **Beans:** You can put beans in many types of recipes. There are many healthful vitamins and minerals in beans that are needed by the cells for improved cellular metabolism. Beans also add fiber to the diet, which helps keep blood sugars and cholesterol under control. You should consume between 20 and 35 grams of fiber daily for good thyroid health.

EXERCISE FOR THYROID HEALTH

You should also boost your metabolism, counteracting the effects of hypothyroidism, through daily exercise. It is best to mix aerobic and anaerobic exercise in order to build muscle and burn calories. Exercise can increase the metabolism for several hours after exercise. If the thyroid level is low, you may not have the strength or stamina for much exercise but whatever you can do in terms of low impact aerobics and lifting weights (or using weight machines) will help your sluggish thyroid do its best.

Fortunately, synthetic thyroid supplements of T4 and T3 are available so you don't have to suffer from the negative effects of low thyroid on your body. Taking the supplements will lower your TSH level, indicating that you are taking the right dose of thyroid supplement. If you are on thyroid supplements, your doctor will measure your TSH level periodically and at least once per year even if you don't have any symptoms of low or high thyroid conditions.

BODY FAT

Women naturally have more body fat than men do. It has to do with the female hormonal milieu and the evolutionary need to have excess body fat for pregnancy and lactation energy sources. Even if you work out with weights and other types of exercises, your body fat measurements will lower but your weight may not move at all. This is because body fat is less dense and takes up more space by volume than muscle tissue. When you exercise to build muscle, you take up less space but weigh the same, because muscle weighs more than fat.

Your Measurements

In measuring your fitness level, it helps to know what your body mass index is. BMI charts are available online, and the formula is bodyweight divided by height (in inches) squared and multiplied by 703.

- Any BMI less than 25 is normal
- BMI between 25 and 29 means you are overweight
- BMI of 30 or greater means you are obese

The problem with weight measurements and the calculation of the BMI is that these measures do not indicate how much body fat you actually have.

An active woman with an increased percentage of muscle when compared to fat may see a higher rating on the BMI scale simply because muscle weighs more than fat. In the same way, a normal BMI doesn't mean you don't have too much body fat.

Belly fat is especially concerning for a woman's health.

Metabolic Syndrome

Women who have extra body fat in the mid- to upper abdominal area have an increased risk of metabolic syndrome, which is characterized by:

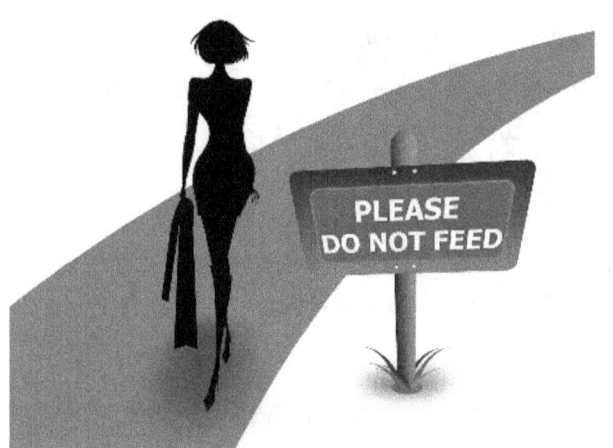

- Abdominal fat
- Diabetes
- Elevated triglycerides
- Low HDL (good cholesterol)
- Increased risk of heart disease

When the body fat is located in the thighs and buttocks, there is a lesser chance of having metabolic syndrome. Extra body fat in the hips increases the risk of developing a deep vein thrombosis in the lower legs, which can become a pulmonary embolism if the clot in the calf breaks off and travels to the lungs. This can be life threatening.

Belly Fat And Life Expectancy

In a study published by the journal Mayo Clinic Proceedings, researchers analyzed data from 11 studies that included more than 600,000 subjects around the world. The results showed that those with the largest waist circumferences were at increased risks of death at a younger age and dying from conditions such as heart disease, cancer, and lung problems. The study showed:

Women with waists of 37" or more had an 80% higher risk of death than those with waists of 27" or less. This equated to a 5-year lower life expectancy after the age of 40.

The Larger The Waist, The Greater The Risk: For every 2 inches of increased waist circumference the risk of death increased by 9% in women. This link between belly fat and increased risk of death was evident *even* in those who had a healthy BMI (an estimate of body fat based on height and weight.

IDEAL BODY FAT

Women should ideally have 16-25% body fat by weight. Even heavy body builders who are female will have more body fat than men will.

Levels less than 15% are just as dangerous as high levels of body fat. Body fat percentages of less than 3% are considered not compatible with life in women.

If you are exercising to lose body, fat but maintain at least a 15% ratio.

Women who are top athletes have a 15-20% body fat, while women who are just fit have body fat percentages of between 21-24% body fat.

An acceptable body fat percentage in women is up to 32%. Overweight and over-fat women have more than 33% body fat.

MEASURING BODY FAT

There are three different ways to measure body fat:

- The first is caliper testing, which measures the fat content under the skin. It has a 3% margin of error. This is the most common tool used in gyms by personal trainers to measure body fat in their clients.
- Body fat scales can be purchased for up to $300 for home use that measures the resistance of the body using an electric current. It also has a 3% of error.
- Underwater (hydrostatic) testing is cheap, usually done at research institutions and has a 1.5% margin of error.

A better way to keep track of your body fat without machines or tests is to look to see how your clothes fit. If you are leaner, your clothes will become looser. Pay attention to your workout and see if you can perform more reps and sets at higher weights than you did when you first began to work out. If you are fit and have a low percentage of body fat, you will have more stamina and energy.

Exercise To Lose Body Fat

When you work out to gain muscle mass and lose fat, you will burn more calories. This is because more calories are burned by muscle tissue than fatty tissue so you may continue to lose weight even if you don't change your diet. Women tend, however, to have areas of the body, which store fat, even when you exercise.

The most common areas of fat storage in women are:

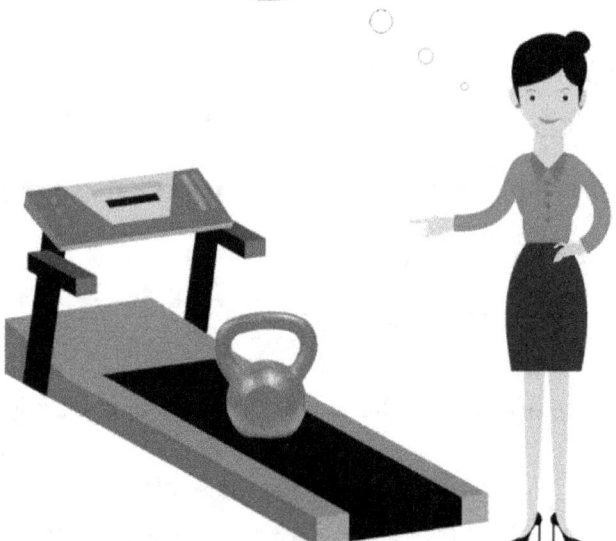

- Lower Abdomen
- Buttocks
- Thighs

This is what gives women their curves; it is very hard to get rid of fat in these locations, even with strenuous or targeted exercise.

Contrary to popular belief, you cannot "choose" where to lose your body fat.
Even if you do sit-ups all the time, the fat is lost throughout the body but you will have an increase in muscle definition in the abdominal area.

Keep your body fat percentage as low as you can through a combination of proper diet, strength training, and aerobic training.

Eat several small meals per day rather than three large meals in support of boosting metabolism for steady calorie burning throughout the day and expect a slow and steady loss of body fat.

CELLULITE

Having cellulite doesn't mean you have a disease or a serious medication. It is only the normal and natural deposition of fat underneath the skin, particularly in the buttocks and thighs. Cellulite fat looks the way it does because it is trapped within connective tissue pockets that make the cellulite look lumpy.

Cellulite isn't dangerous or harmful; it just looks unsightly so that those who get it, particularly women, want to get rid of it so the buttocks and thighs look smoother.

Cellulite tends to happen more in people who are overweight but it can occur in thinner people, too.

Cellulite Is A Common Problem

Sometimes, weight loss can improve the appearance of cellulite but it can't get rid of it altogether. There are many treatments out there for the management of cellulite, many of which don't actually work.

RISK FACTORS

Some people are more prone to getting cellulite than others. Here are some of the risk factors for the condition:

- Slow metabolism, which allows for increased fatty deposits in the thighs and buttocks
- Poor diet that is high in fat or that allows food to turn into fat more readily
- A lack of exercise, which tends to result in increased weight
- Hormones, which is probably why women get cellulite more often than men
- Elevated total body fat
- Dehydration, which makes the fat more visible inside the connective tissue pockets
- Cellulite is more obvious on light colored skin, which is why tanning or using self-tanner helps reduce its appearance

Cellulite does not need to be treated unless you want to look better while wearing shorts or a swimming suit. There are treatments you can do yourself at home and treatments that must be done in a physician's office or hospital.

Creams

The home treatments often involve the application of creams that are supposed to reduce the appearance of cellulite. Many of these creams are made by manufacturers that claim the cream melts or dissolves fat so that the skin is smoother.

A common ingredient in cellulite creams is aminophylline, which is a prescription medication normally used for the management of asthma. While these creams are popular, there are no research studies proving that they actually work on cellulite at all. You would do better to try to lose some weight to decrease the deposition of fat in the tissues, thereby decreasing the appearance of cellulite.

Other creams claim to reduce the appearance of cellulite. One such treatment involves the use of 0.3% retinol cream. This is applied to the affected areas morning and night (twice daily) so that, after about six months, the appearance of cellulite is lessened.

In fact, the creams for cellulite can be dangerous. Aminophylline narrows the blood vessels, dehydrating the skin and messing up the circulatory system in patients who already have circulation difficulties. Allergies, including anaphylaxis, can result from the application of creams containing aminophylline and, when the skin is dehydrated, the connective tissue pockets can become more prominent, making cellulite look worse.

Liposuction

Another treatment for cellulite is liposuction. In liposuction, you undergo surgery that uses a suction trocar placed within fatty tissue, sucking out the fat. The problem is that it doesn't suck out the connective tissue pockets and they can actually look more prominent after the fatty tissue has been sucked out of them.

There is a newer form of liposuction that makes use of laser to increase collagen and tighten the skin. This combined treatment does a lot to help cellulite look better, even if the results are not always permanent.

Mesotherapy

One can undergo mesotherapy, which is a treatment for cellulitis originally performed only in Europe. It is generally used to reduce the pain of inflammation in certain skin diseases but has also been found to help reduce the appearance of cellulite through the injection of amino acids, enzymes, minerals, and vitamins. There is evidence to suggest that it mildly improves cellulite in some people but it can result in an irregular contour of the thighs, swelling at the injection site and infection secondary to injecting substances beneath the skin.

Massage

Massage therapy and other health spa treatments may temporarily reduce the dimpling of the skin seen in cellulite. They do nothing, however, to remove the cellulite from the tissues and the result is extremely temporary and probably due to removal of edema fluid in and around the connective tissue pockets.

Laser Therapy

Laser treatment has recently been approved by the US FDA. This uses a special laser device in a doctor's or cosmetologist's office that melts fat beneath the skin and dissolves the fibrous bands that make up the connective tissue pockets in cellulite formation. Laser stimulates collagen, which can make the skin and underlying tissues thicker.

Infrared light-emitting diodes or LED lights can emit various wavelengths of light, some of which are known to shrink fatty tissue. LED lights are used along with special rollers and suction devices that are designed to soften the tough connective tissue bands that make cellulite lumpier in appearance.

Radiofrequency Therapy

Radiofrequency therapy is another newer form of cellulite treatment. It uses radiofrequency waves along with deep tissue massage at the deeper layers of the tissue to treat cellulite. There is evidence that the use of lasers, radiofrequency technology, and LED treatments can improve the appearance of cellulite for up to six months. After that, the treatments need to be repeated on a regular basis to continue to deliver any results worth noticing.

Exercise

Exercise can reduce the appearance of cellulite, even if you don't lose any weight. Exercise includes both aerobic an anaerobic forms of exercises that tighten the muscles and mobilize fat.

Eating a healthy diet filled with vegetables, fruits and fiber rich foods will help control your weight and decrease the percentage of weight in your body that is due to fat.

A Fact Of Life

Cellulite is basically an unpleasant fact of life, particularly in women who have much of their fat deposits stored in the buttocks, hips, and thighs. When fat is stored there, connective tissue bands within the tissue trap the fat into pockets, which form the dimples often seen when there is cellulite.

As you age, the skin is less elastic and thins out, making the dimpling of the skin more obvious. There is no good treatment for cellulite other than having better lifestyles including eating a better diet, losing weight and exercising on a regular basis.

When the muscles of your thighs are strengthened, the cellulite isn't as obvious and people can see your toned muscles instead. Weight lifting using your legs can increase the strength and improve the appearance of the leg muscles. Often this means using special weight machines targeting the lower extremities.

Nothing can make cellulite go away completely. If you are hereditarily prone to cellulite, there is very little you can do to make it go away once it has begun to occur. Keeping your weight down from a young age can greatly improve your chances of not getting cellulite in the first place.

OSTEOPOROSIS

Osteoporosis is relatively common, affecting approximately 200 million women throughout the world. Osteoporosis or "thinning of the bones" causes 8.9 million fractures every year.

Bones are continually breaking down and remodeling themselves using calcium and phosphorus to create new bone. Whenever there is an imbalance between the breakdown of bone and the rebuilding of bone, osteoporosis can develop.

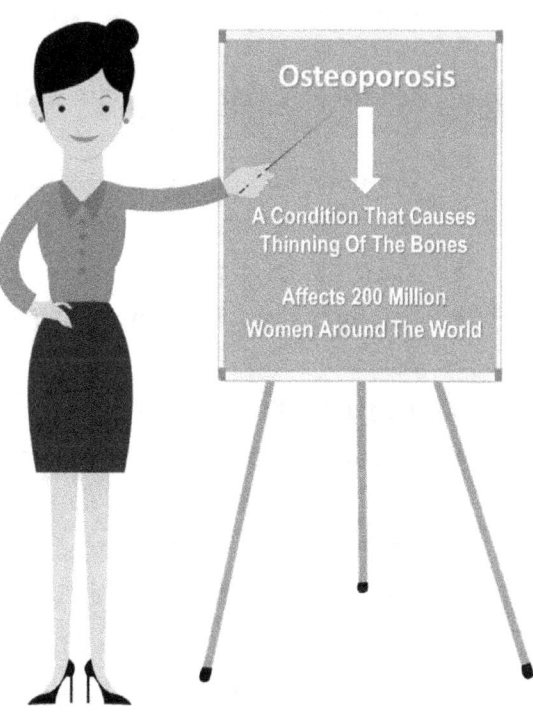

It can cause bones to be so brittle that the act of coughing, walking, or bending over can result in a bony fracture. Most fractures from osteoporosis occur in the hip, spine, or wrist

This condition increases with age, affection 1/10 of women at the age of 60 but 2/3 of women at the age of 90.

Throughout the world, 1 in 3 women older than 50 will have a fracture caused by osteoporosis, while only 1 in 5 men will have an osteoporotic fracture.

SYMPTOMS

There are no symptoms of osteoporosis in the early years. As the disease weakens bones, it can result in the following symptoms:

- Loss of physical height
- Having a stooped posture
- Back pain because of collapsed vertebra
- An increase in fractures, usually caused by little or no trauma

There are several risk factors for developing osteoporosis, some of which are lifestyle factors that are in your control.

Risk Factors For Osteoporosis Include The Following:

- **Gender**: Women are at a higher risk of getting osteoporosis when compared to men.
- **Age:** The risk of osteoporosis increases with age.
- **Race:** Caucasians and those of Asian descent have a higher risk of getting osteoporosis.
- **Family history:** If you have a first-degree relative with osteoporosis, you are at a greater risk.
- **Size of body frame:** People who are small-framed have a greater risk of osteoporosis.
- **Sex hormone levels:** Estrogen is protective against bone loss so that, after menopause when the estrogen levels decrease, women are at risk for getting osteoporosis. Men have decreased levels of testosterone as they age, increasing their osteoporosis risk.
- **Hyperthyroidism:** This condition can increase metabolism, causing more bone loss than bone gain.
- **Parathyroid gland over activity:** A state of increased parathyroid activity can cause a relative loss of bone.
- **Low calcium intake:** You need calcium to build bones so that a low calcium intake can contribute to decreased bone formation and osteoporosis.
- **Anorexia:** Women who do not eat and suffer from anorexia nervosa are at a higher risk of developing osteoporosis. This is partly because of low calcium intake and a decrease in sex hormones.
- **Gastric bypass surgery:** Your risk of malabsorption of calcium is greater after having a gastric bypass surgery.
- **Steroid use:** Those who use steroids like prednisone are interfering with bone rebuilding. Other medications can affect bone density, such as medications for gastric reflux, seizure medication, transplant medications, and chemotherapy.
- **Sedentary lifestyle:** Those who do not exercise much do not stress their bones, which increases bone formation. The result is more bone lost than gained.
- **The use of tobacco:** Those who smoke have a higher incidence of osteoporosis.

DIAGNOSIS

Osteoporosis is identified through a special low-level x-ray test called a DEXA scan. Generally, only the spine, hip and sometimes the wrist are assessed as to bone density. The test is painless and takes less than 30 minutes to complete.

TREATMENT OPTIONS

This condition requires supervised medical care from a qualified doctor. Practicing good habits by increasing your exercise level and eating foods high in calcium can help reduce bone loss. Bone can be gained by taking one of several medications known as bisphosphonates. Some brand name bisphosphonates include Actonel, Boniva, Fosamax, and Reclast. There are oral and injectable forms of bisphosphonates, some of which do not need to be repeated for several months.

Replacing estrogen after menopause can reduce the bone loss that occurs in older women. Estrogen therapy contains its own risks, however; these include an increased risk of breast cancer, heart disease, uterine cancer, and blood clots. Evista (raloxifene) is a drug that mimics estrogen in the body but is safer to take than estrogen alone.

In men, osteoporosis can be averted with testosterone therapy. Testosterone can aid in the increase of bone density in men. Other medications for the treatment of osteoporosis include Prolia, which is injected under the skin at six-month intervals and Forteo, which mimics the parathyroid hormone, PTH.

MENOPAUSE

Menopause is the time in a woman's life when she changes from having regular menstrual cycles from ovaries containing millions of eggs to ovaries that no longer ovulate to release eggs. The ovaries all but shut down so that it makes less of the hormones estrogen, progesterone and testosterone and periods stop.

The average age of a woman at menopause is 51 years of age; however, it can be normal between the ages of 40-59 years. The onset of menopause in a woman under the age of 40 is called "premature ovarian failure."

PERIMENOPAUSE

The perimenopausal years can last for up to five to ten years before the cessation of periods; women experience fluctuations and variations in their periods that can cause irregularity, heavy or light periods, moodiness, and some hot flashes. The average time period of perimenopause is 4 years.

The changes in the ovaries are gradual and the ovaries release less than the normal amount of eggs. As menopause approaches, the drop in estrogen levels is more marked, leading a woman to have menopausal symptoms.

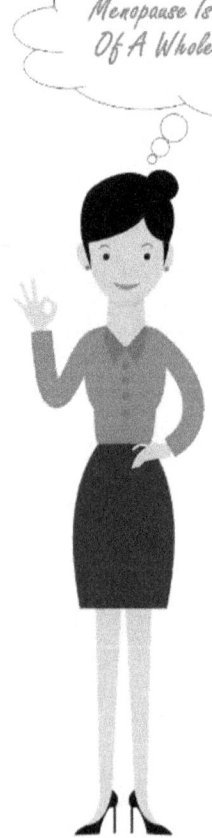

Menopause Is The Beginning Of A Whole New Chapter

The end of perimenopause and the beginning of menopause occurs when a woman has stopped having periods for at least 12 months.

Common symptoms of menopause are related to hormone fluctuations and include the following:

- **Hot flashes:** sudden sensations of flushing or heat in the body, lasting up to several minutes
- **Premenstrual symptoms worsening**
- **Breast tenderness:** caused by a dominance of estrogen
- **Night sweats**
- **Irregular periods:** caused by hormonal fluctuations

- **Decreased libido:** caused by lower hormone levels
- **Fatigue**
- **Urine leakage:** especially when straining, coughing or sneezing
- **Vaginal dryness and pain during intercourse:** caused by decreased levels of estrogen
- **Urinary urgency:** the need to urinate suddenly and without warning
- **Insomnia**
- **Mood swings**

During perimenopause, it is still possible to get pregnant, although the chances are considerably less than in earlier years. Your doctor may run tests to see if you are in menopause; however, hormones fluctuate so greatly that it may be difficult to tell if perimenopause is happening.

The test to see if a woman is approaching menopause is the FSH (follicle stimulating hormone), secreted by the pituitary gland in response to lowered estrogen levels. Sometimes the test is repeated on more than one occasion to get an idea of what the hormone situation is like.

MENOPAUSE

Menopause occurs when a woman has not had a period for at least a year. The ovaries have a significantly decreased their hormone production and the pituitary FSH level is consistently elevated. Menopause means that the protective effect of estrogen on strengthening the bones and on cardiovascular disease is lost so that the woman after menopause has an increased risk of osteoporosis and cardiovascular disease.

Eventually, postmenopausal women have the same risk for heart disease as men, although they do so at a later age.

TREATMENT OPTIONS

Treatment of menopause is directed at reducing the risk of osteoporosis and handling the sometimes intractable symptoms that begin in perimenopause. Osteoporosis treatment involves changing your lifestyle so that you do not smoke, get adequate exercise, eat a healthy diet, and have enough calcium and vitamin D in your system (either through diet or through supplementation). There are medications a woman at risk for osteoporosis can take that stop the loss of bone and help strengthen the bone, as your doctor.

Hormone replacement therapy or HRT involves taking a combination of estrogen and progesterone in order to block symptoms of perimenopause. It can treat the most obvious symptoms of hot flashes, night sweats, and vaginal dryness. If vaginal dryness is the only annoying symptom, estrogen can be given in the form of estrogen vaginal cream.

Women used to take estrogen replacement therapy all the time until an NIH-sponsored study showed an increased risk of breast cancer, stroke, and heart attack in women who took HRT. Now it is given as estrogen and progesterone together for a decreased risk of breast cancer and endometrial cancer in women who know the risks and are suffering greatly from their perimenopausal/menopausal symptoms.

Women can take their hormone therapy orally, through vaginal cream or with transdermal patches or cream, such as is seen when women take specially formulated bioidentical hormones created at compounding pharmacies. Treatment is tapered off when the menopausal symptoms have diminished.

ALTERNATIVE THERAPIES

Various herbs and alternative therapies can help with symptoms of menopause, such as hot flashes and night sweats to improve sleep and therefore alleviate some of the stress that results from these side effects of menopause.

Traditional Chinese Medicine

Tradition Chinese Medicine recommends all natural therapies with the end goal of alleviating all symptoms associated with menopause as they pertain to any individual woman. Instead of a one for all approach, each woman's specific needs are evaluated, and then appropriate remedies are administered. All women are encouraged to maintain a healthy weight, stabilize blood sugar, and alleviate stress and anxiety as much as possible.

- Decreasing stress with the use of yoga, meditation and other natural methods
- Focusing on lifestyle habits that balance the body
- Qigong exercises to increase mental and physical well-being and improving the health of the qi, or life energy within the body
- Eating a diet rich in fish and leafy green vegetable
- Acupuncture is known to alleviate various symptoms
- Herbal supplements to improve kidney and liver energy
- Relaxation

HEART DISEASE

Because women have some protective effect of heart disease due to the presence of female hormones, the risk of heart disease in women is less than in men until they reach menopause, when the risk increases.

Heart disease is defined as being at risk of stroke, heart attack, or peripheral vascular disease because of atherosclerosis. This is when calcium and cholesterol deposits form plaques on arterial walls, eventually blocking the passage of blood through the arteries.

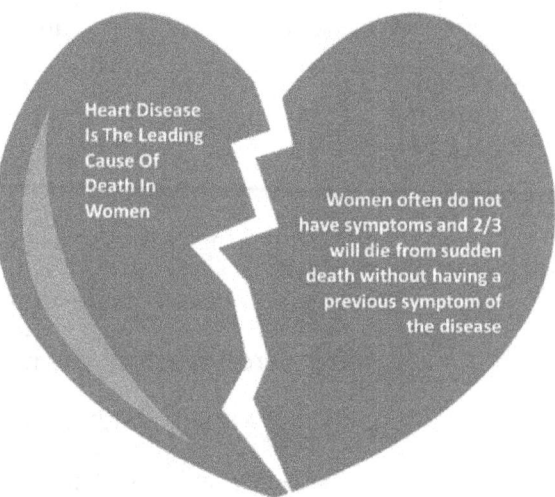

Heart Disease Is The Leading Cause Of Death In Women

Women often do not have symptoms and 2/3 will die from sudden death without having a previous symptom of the disease

The process can occur in any artery but is especially dangerous to the heart, brain, and legs.

STATISTICS IN WOMEN

- Heart disease in women is very common and accounts for 1 in 4 deaths in women. This makes it the leading cause of death in US women.
- In Latina women and American Indian or Asian women, heart disease is the second leading cause of death after cancer.
- About 6% of Caucasian women, 7-8% of African-American women and 5-6% of Mexican American women suffer from coronary artery disease.

Women who have coronary artery disease often do not have symptoms and 2/3 of all women will die from sudden death due to heart disease without having a previous symptom of the disease.

Risk factors for heart disease include: family history, alcoholism, excess stress, smoking, elevated cholesterol levels, diabetes, hypertension, and a sedentary lifestyle, which often leads to obesity.

SYMPTOMS

Many women never show any symptoms, which is one of the main problems associated with this disease in the female population.

If a woman does have symptoms of heart disease, it often manifests itself in angina pain, which is dull or sharp chest pain that radiates to the back, jaw, neck, left arm or upper abdomen.

Angina that comes on with activity and reduces when activity stops is considered "stable angina," while unstable angina is pain that occurs even at rest. Unstable angina is considered more dangerous than stable angina.

Irregular heartbeats can also be symptoms of heart disease in women. If the heart is failing, the woman will experience shortness of breath on exertion and swelling of the legs, ankles, or abdomen.

Other symptoms of heart disease including stroke-like symptoms of weakness or numbness on one side of the body, visual disturbances, and speech difficulty that lasts only a few minutes. If you have any of these symptoms, it is said that you have "transient ischemic attacks" or TIAs, which put you at an increased risk of stroke.

Women who have peripheral vascular disease will often experience "claudication" which is pain in the calf or even the thighs that is brought on by activities such as walking, shiny skin with sparse hair growth in the legs, numbness or tingling of the feet and improvement of symptoms when walking is discontinued. These symptoms can progress to involve open sores of the feet or even gangrene of the lower extremities, necessitating amputation.

PREVENTION

Heart disease is best prevented through lifestyle factors although medications may need to be given. You can decrease

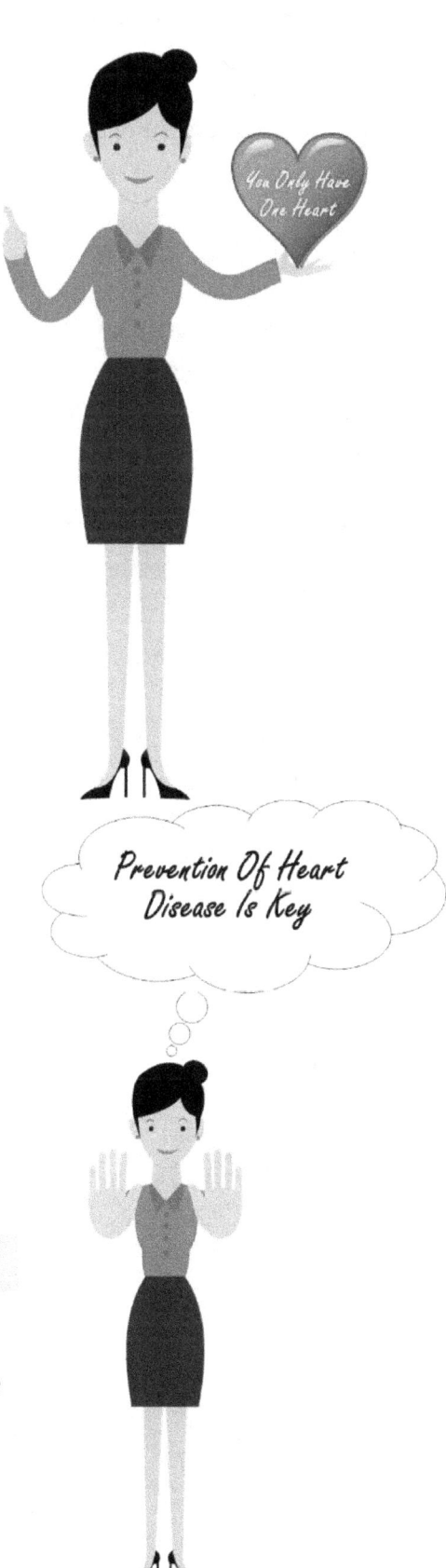

your risk of heart disease by eating a healthy diet filled with fruits, vegetables and whole grains that is low in cholesterol, keeping a normal weight, stopping or never starting smoking, and exercising at least thirty minutes of aerobic exercise per day.

Some women have a family history of heart disease, which usually means they have elevated cholesterol levels and/or hypertension or diabetes.

This might mean taking medications to lower the total and LDL cholesterol, taking medications for high blood pressure, and using medications and diet to keep blood sugars as much as possible in the normal range.

TREATMENT OPTIONS

Various treatments are available for heart disease as prescribed by your doctor. If you already have heart disease, doctors can do procedures such as angioplasty with stent placement, in which a balloon attached to a catheter breaks open the blockage to the coronary artery, using a metal cage called a stent to keep the blockage from reoccurring.

Other procedures include carotid endarterectomy, which removes plaques from the carotid arteries leading to the brain and similar procedures or bypass of the arteries leading to the legs.

BREAST CANCER

Both men and women are at risk for breast cancer, but women shoulder the bulk of this risk.

- According to statistics, 1 out of every 8 women or about 12% will have invasive breast cancer at some point in her life.
- The risk of breast cancer increases with age.
- An estimated 232,000 new diagnoses of invasive breast cancer occur each year. In men, only about 2,350 new cases of breast cancer occur each year with a lifetime risk of approximately 1 out of 1000 men.

Fortunately, the risk of breast cancer is decreasing and began to decrease around the year 2000, which is the time when doctors realized that hormone replacement therapy in menopause increased the risk of breast cancer and stopped prescribing it for most perimenopausal symptoms.

Breast cancer also has a reduced death rate than in previous years with about 40,000 women dying per year from the disease.

The decreased death rate is felt to be due to rigorous screening methods, better awareness of the disease, and better treatment for breast cancer.

1 Out Of Every 8 Women Or About 12% Will Have Invasive Breast Cancer At Some Point In Her Life

SYMPTOMS

When breast cancer is in its earliest form, it generally has no symptoms. This is why a screening mammogram every 1-2 years is recommended, especially as women age past 50.

If breast cancer is allowed to develop, you may notice a lump in your breast on self-examination or a lump in the underarm area that remains after your period. The lumps generally do not hurt although some women experience a prickly sensation in the area of the lump.

One breast can be bigger than the other or there can be a puckering or indentation of the breast due to scar tissue building up around the lump.

Some women experience symptoms similar to a breast infection, with warmth, redness and a pitted surface on one breast. This is a particularly dangerous form of breast cancer.

Paget's disease involves having a scaly rash around the nipple that can signify breast cancer in that breast.

By the time, a breast cancer is able to be felt or when the breast is red and pitted, the chances of metastasis of the breast cancer to the lymph nodes of the underarm or chest wall are high so mammograms, which can detect lumps before they can be felt are important.

RISK FACTORS

Women are naturally at risk for breast cancer when compared to men because of the stimulatory effect of estrogen on breast tissue that occurs during much of a woman's life. Breast cancer is much less common in women under the age of 40 unless there is a strong family history of it in a woman's family.

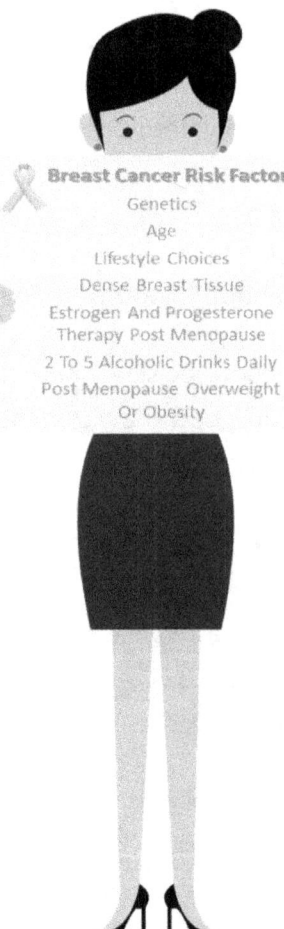

Doctors can screen for some of the genetic risk for breast cancer by doing genetic testing. Mutations of the BRCA1 gene or the BRCA2 gene can be tested for by means of a blood test. Having mutations of these genes put you at a higher risk of breast cancer at a young age. Even if these tests are negative, you could be at a higher risk for breast cancer because not all of the genes responsible for breast cancer have been identified yet.

According to the American Cancer Society, risk factors do not guarantee development of the disease, even in those who may have three or more risk factors.

While some risk factors are beyond our control, such as age and race, others, like lifestyle choices are. All risk factors have varying degrees of risk.

Risk Factors Beyond A Woman's Control

Gender: Breast cancer is 100 times more common among women than men, mainly due to increased estrogen and progesterone hormone levels that promote breast cancer cell growth.

Age: Risk increases with age, and about 1 out of 8 invasive breast cancers occur in women younger than 45, while about 2 out of 3 occur in women age 55 or older.

Race and ethnicity: White women are slightly more likely to develop this disease than African-American women, but African-American women are more likely to die of breast cancer. African American women are more likely to develop the disease in ages 45 or younger than other races. Asian, Hispanic, and Native-American women have lower risks of developing and dying from this disease.

Previous breast cancer: A woman who has or has had cancer in one breast has a 3 to 4 times chance of increased risk for cancer in the other breast.

Dense breast tissue: All breasts are made up of fibrous, glandular, and fatty tissue. Those with dense breast tissue, where there is more glandular and fibrous tissue and less fatty tissue have a 1.2 to 2 times increased risk for breast cancer as compared to those women with average breast density. Breast density is affected by menopausal status, age, pregnancy, genetics and also certain menopause medications, including, hormone therapy.

Benign breast conditions: Certain benign breast conditions slightly elevate risk for breast cancer.

Risk Factors Under A Woman's Control

Having Kids: Women who give birth after the age of 30 have a slightly higher risk, while pregnancies in young ages reduce risk overall, though the effect of pregnancy on risk varies from one type of cancer to another.

Birth Control: Oral contraceptives may result in a slightly higher risk, compared to women who have never used them. Research into this is ongoing, and you should talk with your doctor to ascertain your other breast cancer risks when deciding on birth control pills. DMPA (Depo-Provera®) is an injectable form of the hormone progesterone every three months as a form of birth control. Studies have shown a small risk for breast cancer when DMPA is used.

Overweight Or Obese: Obesity or overweight after menopause increases risks of breast cancer. After menopause, ovaries stop making estrogen and the only estrogen that is produced comes from fat tissue, so the more fat tissue you have the more estrogen is produced thereby increasing risk for breast cancer. Overweight and obesity also correlates with higher blood insulin levels, which has been linked to various cancers.

However, the connection between weight and breast cancer risk is complicated considering that risks increase for women who gained weight as an adult but may not increase for those who were overweight since they were children. Belly fat increases risk more than fat in thighs and hips, as experts believe that fat cells in different parts of the body have different effects.

Exercise: There is evidence that exercise reduces risks of breast cancer. One study showed that as little as 1.25 to 2.5 hours of brisk walking once per week reduces risk by 18% and walking 10 hours per week reduced the risk further.

Hormone Replacement Therapy: Hormone therapy for menopausal symptoms and to prevent osteoporosis uses either a method that includes only estrogen or one that uses a combination of estrogen and progesterone. These treatments use different names, hormone replacement therapy (HRT) post-menopausal hormone therapy (PHT), menopausal hormone therapy (MHT) and estrogen replacement therapy (ERT) or just estrogen therapy (ET).

Studies show that when combined hormone therapy is used it does increase risks for breast cancer and may also increase the chances of dying from breast cancer. There is no indication that ERT (estrogen alone) after menopause increases the risk.

Alcohol Use: Alcohol consumption is clearly linked to an increased risk for developing breast cancer and this risk increases along with the amount that is consumed. When compared to women who do not drink, those who have 1 alcoholic drink a day have a very small risk increase. Those who have 2 to 5 drinks daily suffer 1½ times the risk. Excessive drinking of alcohol also increases risks of developing other types of cancer.

TYPES

There are several different types of breast cancer, including breast cancer in situ, which means there is a localized area of breast cancer that hasn't spread beyond a duct or lobule of the breast tissue.

Invasive breast cancer can be invasive ductal carcinoma, in which the cancerous cells begin in the milk duct and spread out to the fatty tissue of the breast. From there it can metastasize through the blood and lymphatic system. This type accounts for 80% of all invasive breast cancer.

Another common type of breast cancer is infiltrating lobular breast cancer, accounting for 10-15% of all invasive cancer of the breast. This starts with cancerous cells beginning in the milk glands themselves. There are other rarer forms of breast cancer as well.

TREATMENT OPTIONS

Breast cancer treatment continues to advance. Treatment of breast cancer involves surgery, which can mean a lumpectomy, removal of a greater portion of the breast or removal of the entire breast and lymph nodes that carry lymph fluid and cancer cells from the breast.

Chemotherapy and radiation therapy are often done in more advanced cases. Many women are followed up with anti-estrogen medical therapy or other biologic therapy that prevents the growth of any remaining cancer cells. These medications have added a lot to the standards of cancer care in the US. Doctors will tailor a plan for each individual woman, based on her specific needs.

LIFESTYLE DISEASES

Modern society has given us many advantages. We can travel further, work in a wide range of trades and jobs, get better schooling, and manage our day-to-day activities with cell phones and other easy forms of communication. Unfortunately, we also no longer lead simple lives and this has led to a litany of lifestyle related diseases.

Many lifestyle diseases are related to the habits we choose to fight stress. When we forego regular exercise, smoke, use alcohol, sleeping pills, and illicit drugs in order to fight stress, we are contributing to lifestyle diseases that make us sick. Many people engage in these activities, unaware that they are contributing to shortened lives and miserable lives due to illness and disease.

There is a wide variety of illnesses associated with our lifestyles of choice. Reducing stress and improving things like relationships, eating, and exercise all can help reduce these types of problems.

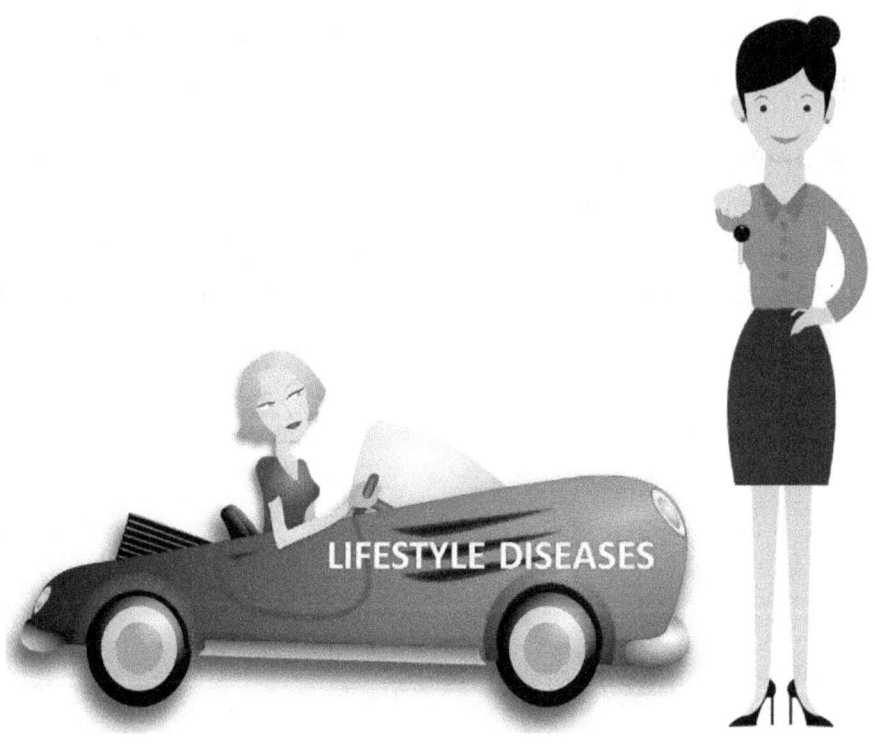

WHAT IS A LIFESTYLE DISEASE

Lifestyle diseases are those that occur mainly as a result of lifestyle choices people make:

- **Certain cancers:** Stress and smoking contribute to the development of lung cancer and reduce the ability of the body to fight off cancer cells. The impact of stress on cancers is not well known but it is believed to be a contributor to getting cancer.
- **Atherosclerosis:** Lifestyles including being sedentary and smoking can cause us to develop elevated cholesterol and high blood pressure, which cause plaques to build up on our arteries, leading to stroke, heart attacks, and peripheral vascular disease.
- **Alzheimer's disease:** This condition has been linked to mental inactivity and stress. It is caused by changes in the brain that cause plaques and neurofibrillary tangles to crop up in the brain, killing brain cells and decreasing the connections between brain cells.
- **Asthma:** Asthma can be made worse by smoking and exposure to allergens. Stress also contributes to the development of asthma symptoms.
- **Cirrhosis of the liver:** Excess drinking and the use of some illicit drugs can put added stress on our liver that must detoxify any pollutant or anything we put in our bodies that might be dangerous. Alcohol intake, when excessive, can lead to cirrhosis or "fibrosis" of the liver and failure of the liver to be able to do its job.
- **Type 2 diabetes:** This condition is related to elevated blood sugars brought on by stress and a sedentary life style, which contributes to obesity – a common cause of type 2 diabetes. Type 2 diabetes is related to a complex problem of insulin resistance that overworks our pancreas, which puts out insulin that doesn't work very well to control blood sugar levels, therefore increasing our risk of type 2 diabetes.
- **Heart disease:** Heart disease is primarily a function of our lifestyle and is made worse by stressors in our lives, poor eating, smoking, and living a sedentary lifestyle that promotes the deposition of arterial plaques in the heart that results in heart disease, including strokes, peripheral arterial disease, and heart attacks.
- **Metabolic syndrome:** A relatively common but poorly understood lifestyle disease that leads to elevated triglyceride levels, diabetes, truncal obesity, low HDL levels, and an increased risk for heart disease. It can be turned around with weight loss, exercise and eating a healthy diet.
- **Stroke:** Contributors of stroke include high blood pressure, a sedentary lifestyle, and smoking. Stroke involves blockages of the arteries leading to the brain or bleeding on the brain that kills brain cells, leaving us with various neurological deficits.
- **Chronic obstructive pulmonary disease (COPD):** This is a disease of the lungs almost exclusively caused by smoking. When we smoke under stress, we damage invaluable parts of the lungs so that there is chronic difficulty breathing and exercise intolerance.

- **Chronic renal failure:** Our kidneys are responsible for getting rid of waste products of metabolism. Things like chronic high blood pressure or diabetes can lead to chronic renal failure that is generally irreversible.
- **Osteoporosis:** When we don't exercise, we allow for weakness of the bone that leaches calcium and phosphorus from bones. The end result is weak bones at risk for fractures, particularly of the hip and spine due to the effects of gravity or to a fall. Regular exercise and diets high in calcium (or calcium supplementation) can bring about stronger bones. It is easier to prevent osteoporosis through diet and exercise than it is to reverse it once it has already occurred.
- **Obesity:** Obesity is a common lifestyle disease brought on by a lack of exercise and poor eating habits leading to an increase in the number of calories taken in when compared to the amount of calories burned. This excess in calories is turned into fat and makes us obese. Obesity can be reversed by proper diet and exercise on a regular basis.
- **Depression:** Depression and anxiety both can result from excess stressors in our life. Stressors we don't have a handle on can cause us to feel out of control, chronically anxious and depressed by our life situations. Psychotherapy and medications that address the neurochemical changes occurring during stress can help alleviate some of the depressive and anxious symptoms.

The effects of a poor lifestyle can build up over time leading to early onset of the above lifestyle diseases. The elderly are most affected by these conditions because they have been exposed to negative lifestyle situations for a longer period of time.

Those of us who live in the Western world suffer from lifestyle diseases more so than those living in developing countries or in the East, where there is a greater emphasis on stress reduction, healthier eating, and exercise. When East Asian people come to live in the West, they begin many of the abnormal lifestyle habits and eventually suffer the same rate of lifestyle diseases as native Westerners.

CAUSES OF DEATH OVER TIME

Lifestyle diseases have markedly changed death statistics in the US in the last century.

For example, in past times the leading causes of death in the US were diarrheal illnesses, pneumonia, influenza, and tuberculosis. Most people died from communicable diseases and many of these diseases now have vaccinations against them or antibiotic therapy to treat them.

Then things changed and we became more industrialized. Food was more processed from factories rather than being grown in gardens or slaughtered from animals. Food became higher in fat and calories with the advent of the fast food industry. We didn't have to exercise as much because of automobiles and sedentary jobs and lifestyle changes took over, causing different diseases to take place. Things like cancer and heart disease killed fewer people in the early 1900s when compared to now, when cancer and heart diseases are among the highest causes of death.

The fact that we live longer has contributed to the buildup of lifestyle changes over time, as people are living longer because we can treat communicable diseases, degenerative lifestyle diseases have taken their place as leading causes of death.

Only reverting to eating healthier food, increased activity, and less stress can reverse some of these lifestyle diseases so we can live longer and more productive lives. This takes commitment to healthier living in a world surrounded by fast food, and sedentary lifestyles that we cannot afford if we want better health.

DIET AND EXERCISE

Diet: Plant based diets rich in nutrients and healthy fats are recommended by experts in furtherance of disease prevention and overall good health.

Physical Activity: Here are the recommended adult physical activity requirements as per the 2008 Physical Activity Guidelines For Americans:

For Important Health Benefits:

Moderate intensity exercise that includes brisk walking or brisk swimming for at least 2 1/2 hours per week **AND** regular weight training for 2 or more days a week.

OR

Vigorous intensity exercise, such as interval training, or running for 1 hour and 15 minutes each week **AND** regular weight training for 2 days a week.

OR

A mix of both moderate and vigorous exercise **AND** regular weight training for 2 days a week.

For Even Greater Health Benefits:

Older adults need moderate to intense activity 5 hours per week **AND** weight training at least 2 days a week.

OR

Vigorous exercise for 2½ hours per week **AND** regular weight training 2 or more days a week.

OR

A mix of both moderate and vigorous aerobic exercise **AND** regular weight training 2 days weekly.

STRESS

Stress affects women nearly every day. With women in the workforce and caring for families, there are more things to balance and be stressed about. Daily stressors can build up over time and cause chronic stress. This kind of stress is often punctuated by acute stressors, such as financial difficulties, moving, relationship difficulties, or a job loss.

Stress doesn't just affect the brain. Stress acts on the whole body to create illnesses one wouldn't necessarily associate with stress. Stress can lead to the onset of disease and can make diseases you already have much worse.

THE STRESS RESPONSE

There are two "arms" to the stress response, both involving the pituitary gland and the adrenal glands.

Fight Or Flight Response

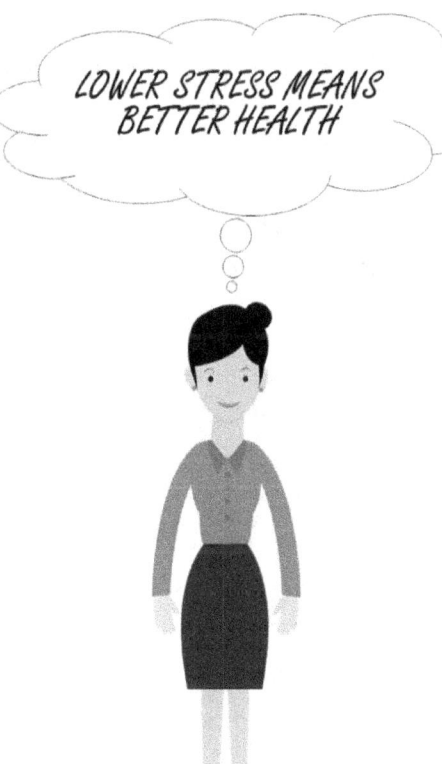

When we are under stress, the brain sends out a signal that reaches the adrenal medulla, which makes epinephrine and norepinephrine. These two stress hormones cause the blood vessels to shut blood away from the core of the body to the brain and muscles in preparation for fighting our imaginary enemies and to think clearer.

Our pupils dilate and our blood pressure and heart rate increase. We feel anxiety and the urge to fight or flee from that, which is perceived, as our stressor.

This is called the "fight or flight" response and is a response ancient man used to fight dangerous animals or run away if fighting wasn't possible. Unfortunately, the fight or flight response does not help us very much in our daily lives as there are few real enemies to fight against.

Stress Hormones

The other arm of the fight or flight response involves the pituitary gland, the hypothalamus and the adrenal cortex. Stress causes the hypothalamus to secrete corticotropin-releasing hormone (CRH), which stimulates the pituitary gland to release ACTH or adrenocorticotropic hormone, which causes cortisol to be released by the pituitary cortex.

Cortisol decreases the functioning of the immune system and an increase in glucose, to be used as fuel in order to fight or flee from enemies. Chronic cortisol stimulation can have a long-standing effect on the immune system, putting us at risk for infections and autoimmune diseases. Cortisol also plays a key role in the development of belly fat.

When our bodies are under a great deal of stress, the adrenal glands become overloaded and can eventually collapse. Adrenal collapse has a set of symptoms all its own and leave us vulnerable to disease.

SYMPTOMS AND EFFECTS OF STRESS

With all of these fluctuations and elevations of stress hormones, there is bound to be chronic effects on the body due to chronic stress. Stress, when not handled appropriately, can lead to generalized effects on your body, your brain and your behavior.

Health problems commonly associated with stress include:

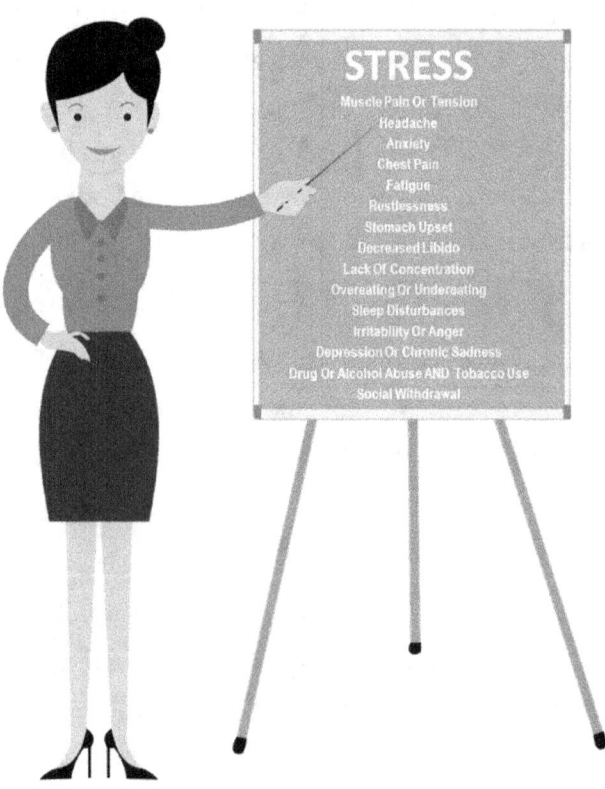

- Muscle pain or tension
- Headache
- Anxiety
- Chest pain
- Fatigue
- Restlessness
- Stomach upset
- Decreased libido
- Lack of concentration
- Overeating or undereating
- Sleep disturbances
- Irritability or anger
- Depression or chronic sadness
- Drug or alcohol abuse
- Social withdrawal

- Tobacco use

While science has not made a direct connection between stress and disease, it is certain that stress plays a key role in diseases like heart disease, high blood pressure, stroke, and diabetes.

Everyone manifests their stress in different ways but having too many of the above symptoms can mean you are under too much stress.

RECOGNIZING STRESS

Not everyone will feel the effects of stress in the same way. Some people can handle a high stress jobs and very busy lifestyles without it manifesting itself physically, mentally or emotionally. For example, those who meditate and practice yoga are better able to cope with daily stress in their lives. Those who practice Tai Chi improve their ability to "let things go" and be more accepting of the world around them, which in turn makes them better able to cope and perceive stress.

When one does not perceive something traditionally viewed as stressful as stress, then they will not suffer the same results as those who do.

It is important to recognize how you view and handle stress, so that you can take action to reduce stress levels.

- Having chronic headaches, body aches or chest pain is a sign you might be under stress.
- The same is true if you develop hypertension or diabetes.
- The effect of stress on the immune system can mean that you cannot fight off infections as well as you normally can and will feel constantly sick or tired.
- When you feel excess anger or irritability or if you feel like you are always sad, dejected, or depressed, this can mean that you are under too much stress.
- In women, stress can manifest itself in abnormalities of the menstrual cycle, leading to abnormal vaginal bleeding or to infertility.

For these reasons, it is important to recognize your stressors and do what you can to eliminate the source of the stress.

DE-STRESSING YOUR LIFE

Sometimes, all it takes is identifying the source of the stress and eliminating it from your life. If your job is giving you excess stress or if the commute to and from work is excessively stressful, it is time to prioritize what is causing you so much stress so you can eliminate it by changing jobs or modifying your existing job to better suit your needs.

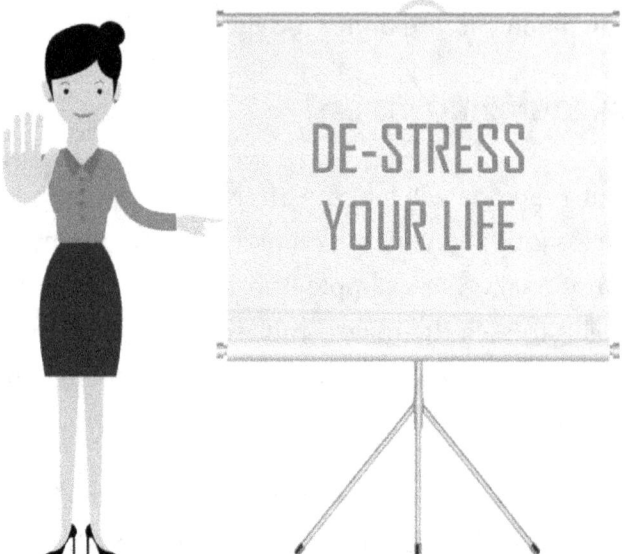

If your stress is due to your family or to a relationship difficulty, you might want to consider family or couple's counseling. This can help you air out your stressors in a safe and controlled manner. It might not only decrease stress but may save a relationship that is in trouble.

Don't be afraid to ask for help. Friends or relatives you have can make your stress better just by listening to your problems or by giving you a hand to lessen the actual stress you are experiencing. Friends or helpful relatives can make all the difference in the world when it comes to accomplishing things in your life that are stressing you out.

MANAGING STRESS

If you can't change some things in your life in order to reduce the stressors, you can train your body to handle stress better. There are techniques and behaviors you can do that will help reduce the fight or flight response in the body, possibly reducing your chance of getting sick because of stress. Some good stress-fighting techniques include the following:

- **Psychotherapy:** Cognitive behavioral therapy or other kind of therapy can help you talk openly about those things that are stressing you. Different types of therapy can help you reframe negative things in your life so that you are thinking about them more positively. It can help you learn relaxation techniques to fight the stress response and can help you problem-solve the stressors in your life.
- **Meditation:** You can learn meditation through a therapist or by purchasing a meditation DVD or CD. Some techniques that work well in meditation include focusing on your breath and heart rate, using your calmer mind to slow your breath down, reduce your heart rate, and lessen your blood pressure. You can breathe while using a mantra such as the commonly

used mantra "ohm," which is a syllable that, when repeated regularly while breathing can soothe the mind and relax your body through progressive muscle relaxation. Guided imagery or visualization works well, too. While meditating, you imagine yourself in a beautiful and peaceful place, such as on a beach, a mountain top or in a forest. Think about the sights, sounds, touch and smells at this location and allow your positive feelings about where you are at in order to calm your mind.

- **Practice yoga:** Yoga is an ancient practice that originated in India and is used by millions of people in the Western world for its plethora of health benefits. During yoga, you practice perfecting specific poses along with concentrating on your breath. Yoga can provide you with increased flexibility, balance, and coordination as well as calm your mind. There are many different types of yoga. Choose a type of yoga that fits best with your physical abilities and that is the most calming for you.

- **Tai chi or qigong:** Ancient martial arts techniques that were adapted for healing from illness or stress, involve going through a series of fluid motions that teach you balance, coordination and focus. People of just about any fitness level can do this type of exercise with positive effects on your body and on feelings of stress.

- **Aerobic exercise:** Any type of regular aerobic exercise will help you deal with stress better. Exercise strengthens the mind and body so that you can feel better about the stressors in your life and can function better in all areas of your life. Exercise releases feel good hormones in the brain that support wellbeing, eliminates nervous energy and improves sleep

FATIGUE

Many women are trying to engage in active and productive lives when really they feel worn out and exhausted. Fatigue can be caused by many different things. If you are suffering from fatigue, it can interfere with your ability to properly perform your daily activities.

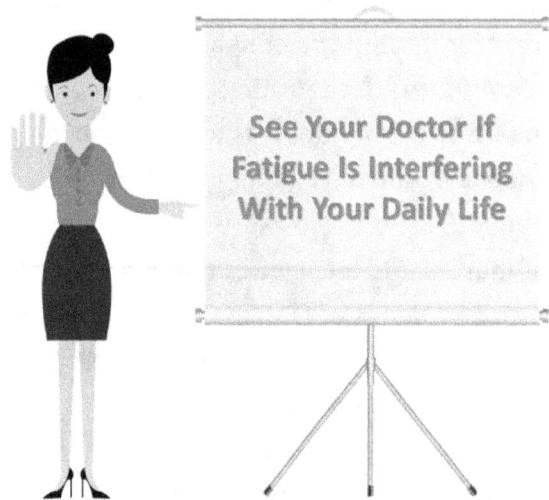

There are many causes of fatigue in women. If you feel you are experiencing fatigue beyond normal, it is worth it to seek the advice of your doctor to help you figure out why you are feeling so dragged out.

TOP CAUSES OF FATIGUE

- **Low thyroid conditions:** The thyroid gland is a small butterfly-shaped gland located in the front of your neck. It produces the hormones that affect your metabolism. If the thyroid gland is overactive or underactive, you can feel tired. You need your thyroid gland to help your cells make use of cellular energy. If the cells cannot use energy appropriately, they will not function properly. Women experience low and high thyroid conditions much more often than men do, although the reason for this is not clear. If the thyroid gland is overactive, you will experience burnout because the cells are over-metabolizing even when it is not necessary. This problem can be treated by destroying any hyperactive thyroid cells and replacing the body with the right amount of thyroid hormone.

- **Heart disease:** Women can be affected by heart disease, particularly after they reach menopause. If you have a family history of heart disease, are overweight, have diabetes, have hypertension, or suffer from elevated cholesterol, you can be at risk for heart disease. When women have heart disease, they don't always have the traditional chest pain that men have but will instead experience shortness of breath and fatigue. Doctors can do a stress test or stress echocardiogram to check to see if your fatigue is related to heart disease.

- **Vitamin D deficiency:** Because we are staying out of the sun more these days and drinking less milk, vitamin D deficiency has become more common. Others are suffering from vitamin D deficiency because their kidneys cannot convert vitamin D to the active form of the vitamin. People who are overweight do not use vitamin D as easily as slim people. Vitamin D deficiency has been linked to chronic fatigue syndrome. See your doctor about having your vitamin D level checked and take a vitamin D supplement if your level is low. You may feel much better when your vitamin D levels are normal.

- **Anemia:** Women have a greater risk of iron deficiency anemia because of regular loss of blood during the menstrual cycle and a lack of iron in the diet to replace the iron lost in the blood. This can lead to chronic fatigue and shortness of breath with exertion. A simple blood test can determine your hemoglobin level to see if it is abnormally low. Multivitamins with iron can replace lost iron so you can feel back to your normal self. Some women need to see a gynecologist if the vaginal bleeding during menses is particularly severe.

- **Sleep apnea:** If you snore or if someone tells you that you have breath-holding spells while sleeping, you may have sleep apnea. People with sleep apnea don't get enough restful sleep at night and the primary symptom is daytime sleepiness. This is because you constantly have to wake up a little during the night in order to get a deep breath. If you suspect you have sleep apnea, have a sleep study to see if you have the disorder and perhaps you will need CPAP therapy, which stands for conditional positive airway pressure. It is a device you wear while asleep that keeps the airways open during sleep time. You will sleep more restfully and will have a better time staying awake during the day.

- **Insomnia:** The stresses of juggling home, work and relationship issues can mean that you don't get the recommended 7-8 hours of sleep per night. When you go too many days without adequate sleep, it begins to take a toll on your daytime level of consciousness. You will begin to have problems with memory, concentration, and mood. The best way to conquer this is to have good nighttime sleep habits and try to get enough sleep every night. See your doctor if you have a serious problem with sleep deprivation and lifestyle measures don't seem to be taking care of the problem.

- **Depression:** Women have two times higher rates of depression as compared to men. Along with depression is fatigue that doesn't seem to get better with sleep. People who suffer from depression are 4 times more likely to be tired than those who aren't depressed. When the depression is treated with therapy and/or medications, you will feel more energy and will find yourself sleeping better.

If fatigue is effecting your day-to-day life, see your doctor, as chronic fatigue can be caused by a variety of medical conditions that may need immediate attention.

If fatigue is something you believe is simply due to lifestyle, making changes can usually help:

- ✓ **Eat a healthier diet:** A diet rich in plant foods can increase energy levels, and junk food does the opposite. Eat a variety of fresh colorful vegetables and lean proteins to increase your energy levels.
- ✓ **Exercise:** Exercise actually creates energy, as opposed to the common belief that it depletes it. A Walk around the block can refresh mind, body, and spirit.
- ✓ **Take short naps:** Cat naps, such as those no more than 15 minutes are very refreshing and really boost energy levels making the day easier to tackle.
- ✓ **Evaluate your schedule:** Are you doing too much? Many "super women" do and pay the price. Consider that if you don't slow down, your body will do it for you.
- ✓ **Reduce Stress:** Stress quickly zaps energy and like anxiety, worry and fear can leave you exhausted, both mentally and physically. Chronic stress incurs long-lived effects so over time you wind up doing less and feeling it more.
- ✓ **Sleep:** Are you getting enough sleep? Experts recommend at least 7 to 8 hours per night.
- ✓ **Increase Magnesium Intake:** Magnesium deficiency may be a cause of fatigue, especially in those who eat a balanced die, but still feel tired. It supports more than 300 biochemical reactions in the body, including breaking down glucose into energy. Women need about 300 milligrams daily, and you can get it from, almonds, hazelnuts or cashews, bran cereal and fish, halibut are especially high in magnesium.
- ✓ **Skip the sugar:** Keeping blood sugars balanced throughout the day keeps the energy flow constant. Sugar and sugary foods cause blood sugar spikes that will give you an initial burst of energy, but because they are too quickly digested by the body that energy is short lived, and you wind up crashing and burning. Conversely, complex carbs, like vegetables, and whole grains are slow digesting carbs that will provide a steady release of fuel to energize you throughout the day with balanced and consistent energy. Try it out for yourself; compare how you feel after eating a Snickers bar versus a bowl of Grape Nuts cereal.
- ✓ **Don't Skip Meals:** Breakfast is very important as it sets the energy stage for the day, and improves mood. Choose complex carbs and lean protein. Studies published in the journal Nutritional Health found that skipping meals leads to more fatigue throughout the day. The body needs fuel to create energy, and its fuel source is food. Choose healthy meals, like fresh raw salads, whole grains, and lean protein in support of energy during the day. Greasy cheeseburgers and fries take a lot more energy to metabolize which leaves you feeling drained and sleepy.

NUTRITION

Today's woman is often struggling to balance work, family, and social obligations all at the same time. Too often, this affects the woman's ability to pay attention to the food she puts into her body and into the bodies of her spouse and family. She doesn't realize that diet can have a great deal of impact on energy levels, mood support, self-esteem, and weight.

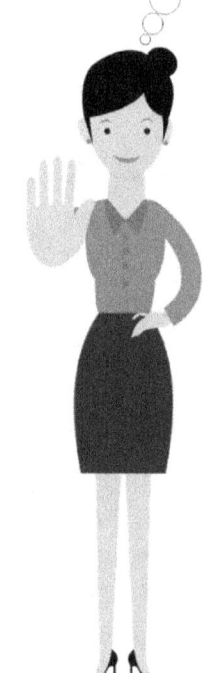

What Do You Put Inside Your Body?

If you are like most women, you are wondering about ways good nutrition can support your body in the healthiest way possible.

Healthy food intake can do a great deal for your overall health, including your mood, your energy level, your menstrual cycle, stress, and even your ability to get pregnant and have a healthy pregnancy.

Women of all ages, really, need to pay attention to their nutritional needs so that, throughout their lifetime, they can remain as healthy as possible.

WHAT IS GOOD NUTRITION?

Good nutrition isn't actually that difficult once you know what foods to eat and what foods to avoid. You should have a well-rounded diet that is based on plant foods.

This means eating fresh fruits and vegetables, whole grains, healthy plant-based fats, and lean protein sources, including lean poultry, beans, and legumes.

You'll find that, when you eat a wide variety of healthy foods, you will have more energy. Many of these foods are low in calories, meaning that you won't become obese and will remain trim and active.

Stay away from highly processed foods, such as those with a great deal of preservatives and animal fats. Processed foods might be faster to make but they tend to be higher in fat and calories than foods you make yourself from fresh ingredients. It means learning a few good recipes and avoiding junk food, sodas, and high fat foods. Meat that has had the bulk of the fat removed or, in the case of poultry, has had the skin removed, can be eaten but shouldn't be the mainstay of your diet.

When in doubt: Food that expires is real whole food. 95% of all food that comes in a box or requires a package is typically not recommended.

HEALTHY FOODS FOR WOMEN

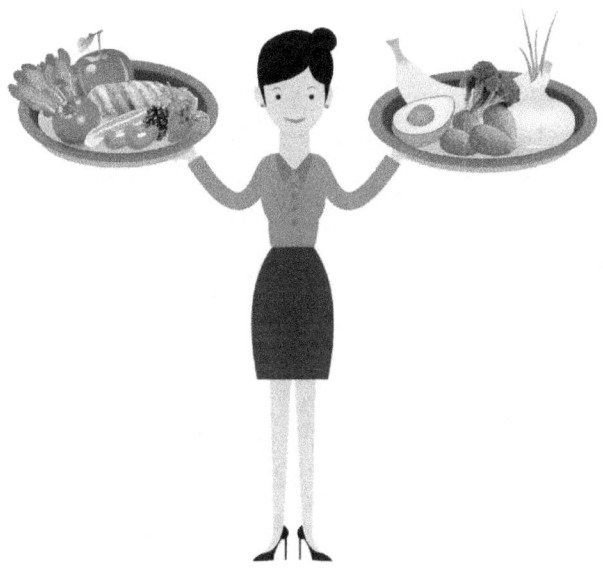

Women have special health concerns that mean they must keep a special outlook toward a healthy diet. Here are a few tips:

- **Eat plant-based foods.** Most plant-based foods are low in calories and fat. These include fruits, leafy vegetables, whole grain breads, beans, and legumes. These foods are high in fiber and keep your blood sugar regulated so that you don't suffer from wide fluctuations in blood glucose. You will keep your weight down with these kinds of foods, which means a lesser risk of many diseases, including heart disease, certain cancers, and diabetes.
- **Get enough calcium.** Women are at higher risk of osteoporosis when compared to men. The amount of calcium in your bones when you are twenty years old plays a role in your getting osteoporosis later in life. Calcium is good for both bones and teeth. You can get your calcium through eating low fat dairy products, and plants like kale, broccoli, Brussels sprouts, beans, and collard greens.
- **Iron is important.** Most women do not get enough iron in their food and women suffer higher risk of iron deficiency, known as anemia than men do. Women also need extra iron because of menstrual loss of blood with each menstrual period. Good sources of

iron include dark poultry meat, lean red meat, spinach, iron-fortified cereal, lentils, and almonds.

- **Decrease caffeine and alcohol in the diet.** This means cutting out alcoholic beverages to less than two drinks per day. High alcohol intake has been linked to osteoporosis. Sodas and coffee both contain caffeine, which can influence your hormone levels and will worsen symptoms of PMS. Sodas contribute to bone loss and increase your risk of osteoporosis. Stick with 1 or less alcoholic beverages per day and drink only one cup of coffee, tea, or soda per day.

- **Keep sugar to a minimum.** Foods high in sugar add empty calories to your diet and increase your risk of diabetes. Avoid things like high-fructose corn syrup, invert sugar, cane juice, corn sweetener, agave nectar, malt sugar, and maltose. Stick to foods that have natural sugars in them like fruits, which make for good desserts after your meal. Stay away from sodas that contain sugar, as these are high in sugar and are empty calories that contribute to weight gain and have no nutritional value whatsoever.

- **Eat a healthy breakfast.** In order to get your metabolism started, you need to eat breakfast every day. Breakfast can involve egg protein, whole grain cereals or whole grain breads and dairy products. Eating breakfast has been known to cut down on snacking later in the day.

- **Eat several small meals daily.** Eating several small meals per day is better than skipping meals or eating three big meals. If you skip too many meals, you get tired and irritable; your metabolic rate goes way down because your body thinks you are starving. Try eating at least 5 to 7 small balanced meals per day and include a snack around 2 pm to ward off low metabolism that typically occurs midway between lunch and dinner.

- **Cut down or eliminate junk food.** Junk food only adds empty calories that are not nutritious for you. Sugary foods can result in mood and energy fluctuations; stick to the complex carbohydrates found in whole fruits, vegetables, and grains like brown rice and quinoa. It takes a few days for the cravings for carbs subside but eventually you will no longer crave junk food and will be happy with healthy food.

- **Eat healthy proteins.** Protein is important for energy and for the function of your cells. Too much protein, especially from animal sources, however, can decrease the calcium in your diet and can put you at risk for osteoporosis. When searching for meat sources of protein, stay away from highly processed meats and instead eat fresh fish, chicken, turkey and low fat dairy products like low or nonfat Greek yogurt. You can get plant-based protein from eating things like nuts, beans, tofu, soy, peas, and seeds.

- **Stick with complex carbs.** Complex carbs such as oatmeal, whole grain breads, bananas, brown rice, and whole-wheat pasta are good sources of fiber and boost your serotonin levels. You will feel fuller longer after a meal with complex carbohydrates when compared to foods high in simple sugars.

COMPLEX VERSUS SIMPLE CARBS

Complex carbohydrates are the right kind of carbs to eat. These carbohydrates are high in fiber and other healthy nutrients. They keep you feeling full longer so you don't eat too much. Your bowel movements will be more regular and soluble fiber will keep your cholesterol down. Fruits, vegetables, and whole grains contain many complex carbohydrates.

These are different from simple carbohydrates that contain no fiber and cause sharp rises in your blood sugar after eating them. The rise and fall of blood sugar will zap you of energy and can contribute to weight gain. Simple carbohydrates are not as filling as complex carbs so you tend to eat more.

To avoid simple carbohydrates, stay away from sugary foods, white flour, and white rice. Many processed sweets are high in simple sugars and should simply be avoided.

GOOD FATS

Unbelievably, having a diet without any fat is not healthy for you. Fat is an important part of cellular structure and you need to have essential fatty acids for many body processes. Healthy fats are necessary for good brain function, healthy skin, food cravings, certain vitamins, and healthy pregnancies. Vitamins A, D, E, and K are only found in foods containing healthy fat.

You should stick to the "good fats," which are monounsaturated or polyunsaturated. These are plant-based fats such as that which is found in canola oil, olive oil, avocados, peanut oil, and many types of nuts and seeds.

Polyunsaturated fats include the omega 3 and omega 6 fatty acids. These are found in certain fatty fish such as tuna, salmon, anchovies, herring, and sardines. Plant sources of polyunsaturated fats include sunflower oil, soybeans, corn, walnuts and flaxseed oil.

Bad fats include saturated fats and trans fat. You can find saturated fats in animal fats, including milk that has not been de-fatted. Trans fats are found in baked goods, shortening, crackers, cookies, snack foods, and other processed foods that are labelled as having "partially hydrogenated fats."

DEPRESSION

Depression is a unique health concern for women. The incidence of depression is two times higher in women than in men.

It is believed that about 1 in 8 women will develop the condition at some point in their lives.

No one knows the exact reason for this but hormonal factors may play a significant role. Experts also hypothesize that women are more likely to seek help for mental distress, which skews the statistics.

Women also express depression differently from men. This may be due to social pressures or to an innate difference in the way, women respond to the chemical changes in the brain that cause depression.

Depression can be very serious. Not only does it mean you have an increase in risk of suicide. Depression can affect every aspect of your life, including your work abilities, self-worth, relationships, and your social life.

SIGNS

Women have a collection of symptoms while they are depressed. Not every woman has all the associated symptoms that go along with depression. Even if you have just a few symptoms of depression, you should see your doctor for evaluation.

Some common signs of depression include the following:

- Loss of interest in activities you used to take pleasure in
- Depressed mood
- Guilty, hopeless feelings or feeling worthless
- Sleeping too much or too little
- Loss of appetite or an increase/decrease in weight
- Problems concentrating
- Fatigue and lack of energy
- Thinking of death or suicide a lot

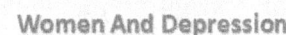

Women And Depression

Depression Is A Unique
Health Concern For Women

Incidence Of Depression Is
Two Times Higher In
Women Than In Men

Hormonal Factors
May Play A Key Role

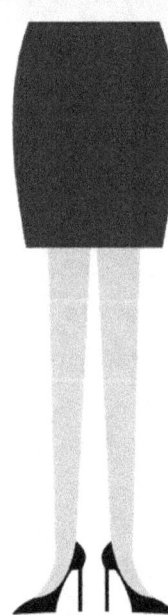

TYPES OF DEPRESSION

- ✓ Women are more likely to suffer from the type of depression that comes on with the darkening of the days in winter called seasonal affective disorder.
- ✓ They also seem to suffer more from atypical symptoms of depression, including sleeping more, gaining weight, and eating more carbohydrates.
- ✓ Women also have a greater incidence of hormonal depression related to low thyroid conditions and premenstrual depression—called premenstrual dysphoric disorder.

Unlike men, women tend to blame themselves more when they are depressed; they also tend to feel more apathetic, sad, and worthless than men do. Anxiety is a big component of depression in women.

They tend to retreat, avoiding conflict, and feel slowed down, while men feel more agitated, restless, and angry while they are depressed.

Women tend to self-medicate their depression with food, although others will self-medicate with alcohol.

BIOLOGICAL CAUSES

Women have more biological reasons to have depression when compared to men. Here are some reasons why the incidence of depression is higher in women than in men:

- **Hormonal fluctuations:** Women have a wide range of female hormones during the menstrual cycle. These hormonal changes can lead to premenstrual syndrome (PMS), which causes irritability, mood swings, fatigue, and bloating in premenstrual women. In some women, the syndrome is so severe that they meet the requirements for PMDD or premenstrual dysphoric disorder. Depressed symptoms are a common part of PMDD.
- **Postpartum depression:** Women go through a huge shift in hormones after pregnancy and some will develop postpartum depression. This type of depression is worse and lasts longer than the typical "baby blues" that almost all women go through for a couple of weeks after giving birth.
- **Pregnancy and Infertility:** Women can be at a higher risk of depression while pregnant or if they have problems getting pregnant. Things like miscarriages, infertility and unwanted pregnancies can yield to depression in susceptible women.
- **Menopause:** There are fluctuations in hormones just prior to and during menopause that can contribute to depression, which seems to be especially prevalent during these years. Women who have a history of depression at an earlier age will have a higher likelihood of having depression during the premenopausal years.

- **Chronic illness and other health problems:** Women are at risk for depression when facing disability due to a chronic illness or when they put their bodies through excess stress when trying to quit smoking or trying to lose weight.

PSYCHOLOGICAL CAUSES

Besides hormones, women can go through depression due to psychological causes. Some of these causes include the following:

- **Excess stress:** Women suffer from having the stress of juggling home, relationship, and work issues all at once. This added stress can affect a woman's brain neurochemicals, which can lead to depression.
- **Ruminating:** Women have a natural tendency to focus on and ruminate over issues in their lives. This can lead to depressive symptoms that don't go away without therapy and/or medication.
- **Body image problems:** Women tend to have a greater degree of body dissatisfaction, which can lead to things like crash dieting and increased stress. These things can affect the body's hormonal milieu, leading to depression.
- **Social stressors:** Women can become depressed over social problems, such as problems with relationships, family responsibilities, work stressors, financial difficulties, or the loss of a loved one.

DEPRESSION MANAGEMENT

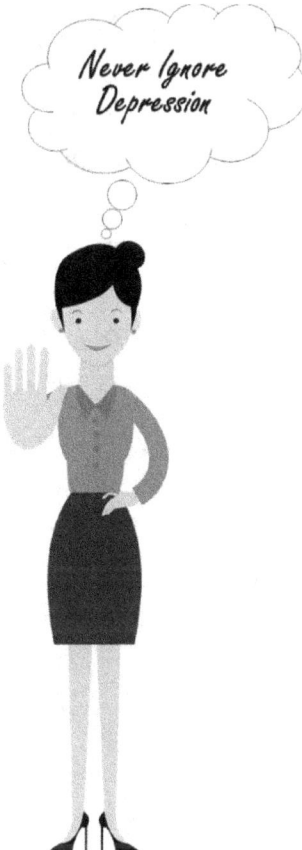

- Some women can improve their depression through psychotherapy, while others will do well on medication alone. A few require both psychotherapy and medication to improve their symptoms.
- Common medications used for depression include selective serotonin reuptake inhibitors or SSRIs. These raise the levels of serotonin in the brain, causing a relief of depressive symptoms. Some common antidepressants include Prozac, Celexa, Paxil, and Lexapro.
- Selective norepinephrine reuptake inhibitors like Wellbutrin will help other women suffering from depression.
- If premenstrual syndrome or PMDD is part of the problem, sometimes the use of birth control pills to help even out the hormones during the menstrual cycle will help the depressive symptoms without the use of other antidepressant medication. On the other hand, some women will have worsening of their symptoms on birth control pills. This is why it is necessary to work with your doctor to try and find the proper balance of hormones and medications that will control the symptoms.

WHAT YOU CAN DO

It is sometimes helpful to consider changing your lifestyle a bit when suffering from depression. Certain lifestyle changes will help depressive symptoms without the use of antidepressants.

Some things you can do include:

- ✓ Get regular exercise at least thirty minutes per day, the exercise you get doesn't have to be strenuous, even a thirty minute walk in the sunshine can improve your mood.
- ✓ Try relaxation methods such as guided visualization, meditation, and yoga will improve mood and decrease depressive symptoms.
- ✓ In the winter, special light boxes can be used at your workplace or while reading that enhance the brain's ability to tolerate the lower light of winter.
- ✓ Be sure to talk to someone about what you're going through. This can be a pastor, therapist, or really good friend. Talking about your problems can help dissipate some of the helplessness you may feel around them.
- ✓ Try to be as social as possible even when you think you can't. Being around people will help prevent rumination.

- ✓ Get at least eight hours of sleep per night. Sleep helps your brain regenerate at nighttime and you have fewer mood symptoms when you get enough sleep.
- ✓ Find something to do that you find is meaningful and that helps you relax. This could mean volunteering or helping others in any way you can. When you have a purpose, you worry less about yourself and focus on more important things in life.
- ✓ Seek help from a family doctor or gynecologist if you feel your symptoms are related to your menstrual cycle. Women who have PMDD often have prolonged periods of depression that are only somewhat better after the onset of the menstrual period. The treatment can involve hormonal therapy or the use of SSRI antidepressants, which are taken throughout the menstrual cycle. There are even herbal remedies that can help with depression related to or unrelated to your period.

AUTOIMMUNE DISEASES

An autoimmune disease is one in which the body makes antibodies against its own tissue, mistaking it for foreign tissue. Cells of the body are targeted for destruction and die off. There are a great many types of autoimmune diseases, some of which are common and some of which are rare.

Types Of Autoimmune Diseases:

- Type 1 diabetes
- Rheumatoid arthritis
- Hashimoto thyroiditis
- Graves' disease
- Systemic lupus erythematosus (lupus)
- Scleroderma
- Sjogren's disease
- Celiac disease
- Guillain-Barre disease
- Psoriasis

STATISTICS ON WOMEN WITH AUTOIMMUNE DISEASE

There are about 50 million people with some sort of autoimmune disease in the US; of those, more than 75% are women.

Taken together, autoimmune diseases account for the 4th most common cause of disability among women.

No one knows why autoimmune diseases occur or why women get the disorders more than men do. Heredity appears to play a role in who gets autoimmune diseases but environmental causes, such as hormones, may also play a role. People can get autoimmune diseases at any time in their life but it is most common among those who are in their childbearing years.

DIAGNOSIS OF AUTOIMMUNE DISEASES

Autoimmune diseases can be difficult to diagnose, especially since they can be rare and often have symptoms that overlap other diseases. If an autoimmune disease is suspected, the doctor orders certain tests, such as the FANA test (fluorescent antinuclear antibody test) and a sedimentation rate (SED rate). These can indicate that an autoimmune disease is going on but cannot tell which kind it is. It is up to the doctor treating you to consider your symptoms in order to diagnose the exact type of autoimmune disease you have. The diagnosis can take months or even years to become clear.

One survey (by the Autoimmune Diseases Association) found that more than 45 percent of women with real autoimmune disease were labeled as having psychosomatic disease or malingering in the early stage of the disease. Another study showed that, in some cases, it can take five different doctors and up to 4 ½ years to make a correct diagnosis.

The diagnosis can be confounded by the fact that autoimmune diseases are inherited as a disease cluster rather than just a single disease. One member of the family may have lupus, while another has Hashimoto's thyroiditis or rheumatoid arthritis. This is why it is important to know if any close family members have any type of autoimmune disease whatsoever. This can lead the doctor to look more closely at an autoimmune disease being the cause of your symptoms.

Women have better immune systems than men do in general. This means they have a better resistance to infection but have a greater risk of having the immune system become hyperactive, causing an autoimmune disease. There may be other factors as to why women have autoimmune diseases more readily but the research specifically involving women with autoimmune diseases just isn't yet available. In addition, different ethnic groups have a greater chance of having some autoimmune diseases and not others. Nine out of ten people with lupus are women and more African-American, Asian, Native American, and Hispanic women seem to have the disease more than Caucasian women do. Exactly why this is the case is unclear.

Autoimmune Diseases As A Whole

More research needs to be done on autoimmune diseases as a whole rather than on specific diseases. All autoimmune diseases have the same basis in the immune system with the differences being which target tissue is involved. More research is also needed to identify triggers to autoimmune diseases in women specifically. Prevention of autoimmune diseases needs to be the focus of more research because, once a person has the autoimmune disease, they have the disease for the rest of their lives.

TREATMENT OPTIONS

Different autoimmune diseases can be treated in similar ways. For example, corticosteroids, which block the immune response, have been found to be helpful in many cases of autoimmune disease. In other diseases, avoiding triggers like gluten in celiac disease are disease-specific. New biologic treatments are available for many different kinds of autoimmune disease. The treatment you receive depends on what kind of autoimmune disease you have as well as on your personal response to the treatments tried.

CONCLUSION

Don't wait for a rainy day to look after your health!

There are many things you can do to ensure that you maintain optimal health and wellbeing well into old age.

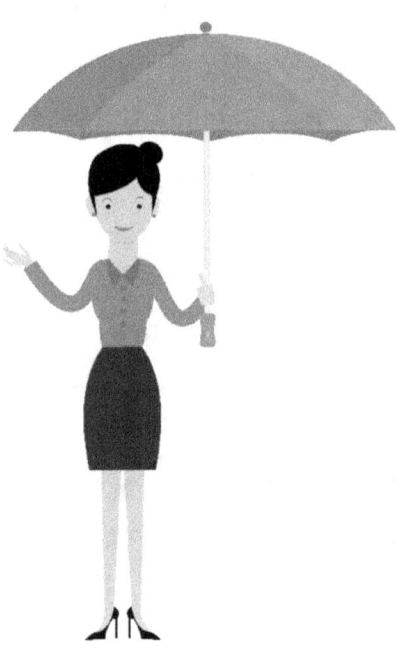

Awareness of your bodily functions and special needs as a woman is the first step.

Action is the second!

When we take care of our bodies, they take care of us. See your doctor regularly for preventative care and look to healthy lifestyle choices to drive your longevity and remain disease free.

Make sure to address stress and fatigue to not only improve your overall quality of life, but also to lower risks for chronic disease that can affect you as you get older.

Last but not least, remember that all of us are responsible for our own good health, and we are worth it!

Stay Well!

"You only live once, but if you do it right, once is enough."
~ Mae West